Re-balance Your Body: 25 Detox Smoothies for Leveling Your Hormones, Flushing Toxins, and Promoting Weight Loss

Disclaimer and Terms of Use: Effort has been made to ensure that the information in this book is accurate and complete, however, the author and the publisher do not warrant the accuracy of the information, text and graphics contained within the book due to the rapidly changing nature of science, research, known and unknown facts and Internet. The Author and the publisher do not hold any responsibility for errors, omissions or contrary interpretation of the subject matter herein. This book is presented solely for motivational and informational purposes only.

Table of Contents

Lemon Aloe Smoothie

Ingredients:
- 1 C coconut water
- ½ avocado
- ½ C aloe vera gel
- ½ lemon, seeded
- ½ lime, seeded
- 1 T honey
- ice
- 1 T flaxseed

Directions:

I.   Start with adding everything into your blender or food processor

II.   Blend everything on medium to high, until well blended

III.   Serve

Watermelon Flower Smoothie

Ingredients:

- ½ C water
- 1 C seeded watermelon
- 1 banana, frozen
- 1 C chopped dandelion greens
- lime juice
- ¼ tsp. cinnamon
- ½ tsp. grated ginger

Directions:

I.   Start with adding everything into your blender or food processor
II. Blend everything on medium to high, until well blended
III. Serve

Tropical Detox

Ingredients:
- ½ C water
- ½ C cilantro
- 1 C pineapple
- ½ C mango
- ½ C kiwi

Directions:

I.   Start with adding everything into your blender or food processor

II.   Blend everything on medium to high, until well blended

III.   Serve

Sour Lemonade Smoothie

Ingredients:
- ½ C water
- ½ C ice
- 1 lemon, seeded
- 1 apple, cored and wedged
- 1 banana
- 1 tsp. coconut oil
- ½ tsp. grated ginger spice

Directions:

I.   Start with adding everything into your blender or food processor
II.   Blend everything on medium to high, until well blended
III.   Serve

Mango Lime Smoothie

Ingredients:
- 1 C coconut water
- ½ avocado
- ½ C cilantro
- 1 C spinach
- 1 C fresh mango, cubed
- lime juice
- ½ tsp. honey

Directions:

I.   Start with adding everything into your blender or food processor

II.   Blend everything on medium to high, until well blended

III.   Serve

Spanish Smoothie

Ingredients:
- 1 C coconut water
- ice
- banana
- ½ C cilantro
- lime juice
- ½ coconut oil
- salt and pepper
- honey
- ½ C pineapple bites

Directions:

I.   Start with adding everything into your blender or food processor
II.   Blend everything on medium to high, until well blended
III. Serve

Four Seasons Smoothie

Ingredients:
- 1 C spring water
- ½ C lemon
- 1 C kale
- 1 C dandelion greens
- 1 apple, cored
- 1 pear, cored
- ½ tsp. ginger powder
- ¼ tsp. cayenne pepper
- 2 C arugula

Directions:

I.   Start with adding everything into your blender or food processor
II.   Blend everything on medium to high, until well blended
III.   Serve

Cranberry Cleanser

Ingredients:
- 1 C water
- 1/2 C cranberries
- 1 apple, peeled and cored
- 1/2 lemon, seeded
- 1/3 avocado
- 1/2 tsp. nutmeg
- 1/2 C blackberries

Directions:

I.   Start with adding everything into your blender or food processor
II.   Blend everything on medium to high, until well blended
III.   Serve

Ginger Watermelon

Ingredients:
- 2 C seeded watermelon
- 1 T ginger powder
- lime juice
- ½ C mixed berries

Directions:

I.   Start with adding everything into your blender or food processor
II.   Blend everything on medium to high, until well blended
III. Serve

The Lemon Lime

Ingredients:

- 1 C coconut water
- ½ lemon, seeded and peeled
- ½ lime, seeded and peeled
- 1 banana
- 1 T honey
- ½ T ginger powder
- ½ C mixed berries

Directions:

I.   Start with adding everything into your blender or food processor
II. Blend everything on medium to high, until well blended
III. Serve

Berry Smoothie

Ingredients:
- 1 C raspberries
- ¾ C almond milk
- ¼ C cherries, pitted
- 1 ½ T honey
- 2 tsp. grated ginger, fresh
- 1 tsp. ground flaxseed

Directions:

I. Start with adding everything into your blender or food processor
II. Blend everything on medium to high, until well blended
III. Serve

CranVanilla Smoothie

Ingredients:

- 1 ½ C almond milk
- 1 C greek yogurt
- 1C berries
- ice
- 1T cranberry powder
- 1 tsp vanilla

Directions:

I.   Start with adding everything into your blender or food processor
II.   Blend everything on medium to high, until well blended
III.   Serve

Banana Pineapple

Ingredients:
- 1 C banana
- 1 C pineapple
- 2 C spinach
- 1 C coconut water

Directions:

I.   Start with adding everything into your blender or food processor

II.   Blend everything on medium to high, until well blended

III.   Serve

Breakfast Smoothie

Ingredients:

- 1 C soy milk
- ½ avocado, chopped
- ½ T nutritional yeast
- 1 ½ T syrup
- ½ tsp. ground flaxseed
- ½ tsp. vanilla
- ¼ tsp. ground cinnamon

Directions:

I.   Start with adding everything into your blender or food processor
II.   Blend everything on medium to high, until well blended
III. Serve

Green Pie

Ingredients:
- 1 tsp. pumpkin pie
- spice
- ¼ tsp. cinnamon
- ¼ tsp. vanilla
- 1 tsp. maple syrup
- ice

Directions:

I.   Start with adding everything into your blender or food processor
II.   Blend everything on medium to high, until well blended
III. Serve

Luck of the Irish Detox

Ingredients:
- 1 C spinach
- 1 C kale
- 1 avocado
- ½ green apple, cored
- 1 ¼ C orange juice
- 2 T agave
- 1 C ice
- ¼ water
- ½ tsp. Vanilla

Directions:

I.   Start with adding everything into your blender or food processor
II.   Blend everything on medium to high, until well blended
III.   Serve

Ingredients:
- 1-2 bananas
- 1 C Spinach
- 1 ½ C almond milk
- ¼ C yogurt
- Stevia to taste

Directions:

I. Start with adding everything into your blender or food processor
II. Blend everything on medium to high, until well blended
III. Serve

The Pina

Ingredients:
- ¾ C canned coconut milk
- ¾ pineapple, chunked
- banana
- 1 T honey
- 1 tsp. lime juice
- salt

Directions:

I.   Start with adding everything into your blender or food processor

II.   Blend everything on medium to high, until well blended

III.   Serve

Blue Lemon Smoothie

Ingredients:
- ¼ C stewed peaches
- ½ C blueberries—frozen preferred
- 1 T lemon juice
- ¾ C almond milk
- ice
- Stevia to taste

Directions:

I.   Start with adding everything into your blender or food processor
II.   Blend everything on medium to high, until well blended
III. Serve

Chocolate Avocado Smoothie

Ingredients:

- ½ avocado
- 2 T cocoa powder
- 1 banana
- ½ C greek yogurt
- 2 T almond milk

Directions:

I.   Start with adding everything into your blender or food processor
II. Blend everything on medium to high, until well blended
III. Serve

Power Basil

Ingredients:

- 2 bananas
- 2 C blueberries
- basil
- 2 T nut butter
- 1 T maple syrup
- 2 T ground flaxseed
- 2 C almond milk

Directions:

I. Start with adding everything into your blender or food processor
II. Blend everything on medium to high, until well blended
III. Serve

Squash Smoothie

Ingredients:
- 2 C butternut squash
- 2 apples, cored
- 1 banana
- 1 C coconut milk
- 2 T peanut butter
- 1 ½ tsp. cinnamon
- ½ tsp. ginger powder

Directions:

I.   Start with adding everything into your blender or food processor
II.   Blend everything on medium to high, until well blended
III.   Serve

Green Coffee

Ingredients:
- 3 T walnuts, rushed
- 2 T oats
- ¾ C almond milk
- ½ T espresso or mocha
- Stevia
- ½ tsp. vanilla
- 1 tsp. maple
- 2 dates
- ice

Directions:

I.   Start with adding everything into your blender or food processor
II.   Blend everything on medium to high, until well blended
III.   Serve

Cherry Almonds

Ingredients:
- 1 C almond milk
- 1 C cherries
- 2 T honey
- 1 tsp. cinnamon
- ½ tsp. almond extract
- 1 T coconut oil

Directions:

I.   Start with adding everything into your blender or food processor
II.   Blend everything on medium to high, until well blended
III.   Serve

Mango Smoothie

Ingredients:
- 1 mango, peeled, sliced
- 1 banana, peeled, sliced
- 1 C almond milk
- 1/3 C orange juice
- 1/3 C Greek yogurt
- lemon or lime juice

Directions:

I.   Start with adding everything into your blender or food processor
II. Blend everything on medium to high, until well blended
III. Serve